The Companion Guide to
# The **Road** to **Perfect Health**

*How Probiotics Balance Your Gut and Heal Your Body*

**BRENDA WATSON**, C.N.C.

**Renew Life Press and Information Services**
198 Alt.19 South
Palm Harbor, FL 34683
1-800-830-4778

# Contents

# Preface

## by Brenda Watson, C.N.C.

I grew up like any average Southern girl. On the outside, it didn't seem like I was any different from the rest of the kids I went to school with, but inside I was weighed down by a terrible problem: I couldn't go to the bathroom.

I mean I did occasionally, but it was just that—occasionally. And each time I did have a bowel movement it was a painful task with little to show for it. Soon I started to avoid going to the bathroom altogether, which only made things worse.

Nobody knew it, but because I couldn't get this stuff out of my body, I was literally poisoning myself. The toxins building up inside me gave me violent migraines that started in middle school, along with bone-wearying fatigue and frequent infections that just seemed to pile up on each other.

By the time I reached my 20s I had had enough; I went on a mission to research and solve my problems on my own . . . and I did.

More than three decades later, not only have I reclaimed my body and my health, but I have helped thousands of other people do the same—first through establishing five digestive care clinics and working hands-on with patients, then through developing my own natural health formulations based on what I had learned, and eventually through the process of writing several books, including a *New York Times* best-seller, as well as sharing my message through my national television specials and personal appearances.

When I was struggling with digestive problems, it was a dark time in my life. Everything was affected by it, but since I've taken back control of my body and my health, everything has changed. Now I'm on a mission to make sure you get the same chance to break free and discover the path to vibrant health and energy for life. Visit my website, www.brendawatson.com, for my latest updates.

# Introduction

As a natural health practitioner for over twenty years specializing in digestive health, I can tell you that poop is my passion! The subject may seem taboo, but I'm here to spread the word that as a nation, we've got serious digestive and elimination problems. Irritable bowel syndrome (IBS) is the most common chronic medical condition in the Western world, with 15 to 20 percent of all adolescents and adults suffering from it. It's time to get over our embarrassment about the subject and start talking about poop!

Constipation is one of the most common gastrointestinal complaints in the U.S. Each year, more than four million Americans experience frequent constipation requiring a doctor's visit. This underestimates the true prevalence, however, since Americans spend over $725 million self-treating their constipation with over-the-counter laxatives, likely never visiting a doctor. Constipation is traditionally defined as less than three bowel movements per week, but most natural health practitioners consider less than one bowel movement per day to be an indication of constipation.

Heartburn, also known as acid reflux, is another common digestive disorder affecting over sixty million Americans at least once a month, and about 15 million Americans on a daily basis. Acid reflux episodes occurring two or more times per week indicate a condition known as gastroesophageal reflux disease (GERD). If the underlying causes of GERD are not resolved, more serious conditions, like Barrett's esophagus or even esophageal cancer, may develop.

In addition to the many gastrointestinal conditions affecting Americans today, we are faced with an epidemic of cardiovascular disease, mood disorders like anxiety and depression, autoimmune conditions like type 1 diabetes and multiple sclerosis, and allergic conditions like asthma and eczema. You might think that these conditions have nothing to do with the gut, but you're wrong. Though the digestive system seems to be self-contained, the gut is the root and core of our overall health. In the gut, food is broken down into nutrients our body absorbs and uses for every function of the body. The gut is our first

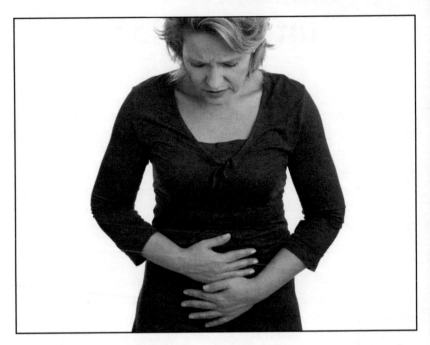

line of defense against pathogens and infections. The gut protects us against environmental toxins that can leak into the bloodstream. The gut is home to 80 percent of our immune system. I'm here to help you connect the dots between gut health and the health of the rest of your body.

You might be wondering how the digestive system can have such a big impact on your health. I have one word for you: BACTERIA. We've been taught that bacteria are bad, something we need to get rid of, and stay away from. But the truth is our bodies are filled with bacteria. About 100 trillion bacteria cells reside in your gut—that's ten times the amount of cells that make up your entire body! And those bacteria have over 100 times the genes that make up your own human genome. According to Thomas Insel, M.D., Director of the National Institute of Mental Health (NIMH), "We are, in fact, 'super-organisms' made up of thousands of species."

The bacteria naturally found in the digestive tract not only serve to protect and maintain digestive health, but also the health of the whole body. These beneficial bacteria are known as probiotics. I call this protective system your "GPS": your very own Gut Protection System. Your GPS works hard to protect your health, but it can encounter many obstacles along the way.

The beneficial gut flora can be destroyed, bringing your GPS out of balance. Poor diet, stress, medications like antibiotics, and even age can all affect your gut bacterial balance. When this balance is upset, harmful bacteria can gain the upper hand, creating digestive disturbances that lead to many serious health problems.

You have the power to balance your gut and heal your body. Consuming probiotics from supplements and food will help to replenish the good bacteria and get your GPS back on track. For over 100 years scientists have recognized the beneficial effects of probiotics, mostly the species of Lactobacillus and Bifidobacterium. A healthy balance of these bacteria in the gut can bring about good health.

In this booklet, you will learn how your GPS works to keep your health on track. Then, you will learn what factors can pull your GPS off track and how to avoid those detours so you can live a healthy life. Next, I'll tell you all about probiotics and how they work. You'll learn what to look for when selecting a probiotic product. After that, I'll connect the dots between digestive health and total body health, highlighting the beneficial role probiotics play in bringing your GPS back into balance. Finally, you'll find answers to frequently asked questions about probiotics and health. So get over your shyness about talking poop, and let's get your GPS back on track.

# PROBIOTICS
## & HEALTH CONDITIONS

Countless studies have shown a balanced gut to be directly or indirectly helpful in broad health conditions and specific digestive conditions including:

✓ Constipation
✓ Heartburn/GERD
✓ Irritable Bowel Syndrome
✓ Gas/Bloating/Indigestion
✓ Antibiotic-Associated Diarrhea
✓ Traveler's Diarrhea & Viral Diarrhea

✓ Muscle/Joint Pains
✓ Weight Gain/Obesity
✓ Fatigue/Energy Levels
✓ Immune System Issues
✓ High Cholesterol
✓ Skin Problems
✓ Allergies

# CHAPTER ONE

# Your Body's Own "GPS"
## (Gut Protection System)

Your digestive tract, also known as the gastrointestinal (GI) tract, is responsible for moving food from the mouth to the stomach, and then through the small and large intestines. Inside the GI tract food is broken down and digested so that nutrients can be absorbed and utilized by the body. These basic functions are what most people typically think as the only functions of the digestive tract. But there is far more going on down there than simply the food processing of digestion.

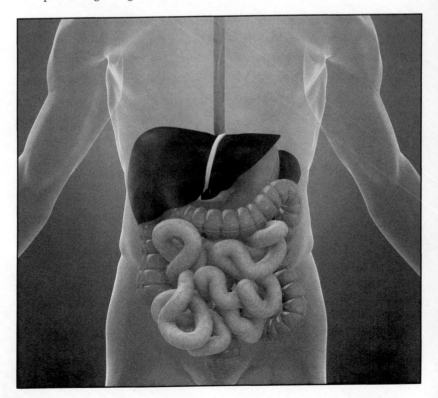

The entire digestive tract is actually colonized by bacteria. As a matter of fact, you have ten times more bacteria cells in your gut than cells making up your entire body. There are over 1,000 (some experts say as many as 10,000 or more) species of bacteria in your gut. Collectively, these gut bacteria weigh about four pounds—that's as heavy as a brick. What's more, there are over 100 times the genes that make up bacteria as there are in your own human genome.[1] This suggests that our bacterial genome may have more impact on our health than our own genes. In fact, the gut microbiota is considered by some experts to be an organ itself because its functions are essential for survival.[2]

But wait—before you get worried about all these bacteria, let's clarify. There are three types of bacteria: beneficial, neutral, and harmful. The majority of bacteria in your gut should be the beneficial, or friendly, bacteria—otherwise known as probiotics. Probiotics are your Gut Protection System, or "GPS." The balance of bacteria in your gut determines the health of your digestive system, and, in turn, the health of your entire body.

**Your GPS works in three main ways:**

1. It produces substances that neutralize harmful bacteria;
2. Protects the intestinal lining and improves the balance of good to bad bacteria in the gut by "crowding out" bad bacteria; and
3. Influences the immune system so that it responds appropriately to invaders, such as harmful organisms, toxins, and even food.

The complex community of gut bacteria, also known as the gut flora or microbiota, is unique to each individual—everyone has their own gut microbial fingerprint, which begins developing at birth. Major differences in gut bacteria are seen between infants born vaginally and those born by Cesarean.

# RULES OF L&B

Specific strains of probiotics benefit certain parts of the digestive tract more than others. **Lactobacillus** strains work better in the small intestine, and **Bifidobacterium** strains work better in the colon (large intestine). A good rule of thumb is to look for a multi-strain probiotic with lots of L's for the little (small) intestine, and B's for the big (large) intestine. For more information visit www.ultimateflora.com

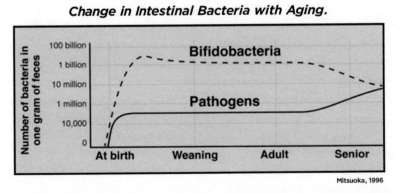

**Change in Intestinal Bacteria with Aging.**

Mitsuoka, 1996

This is because the mother's vaginal tract is also colonized by bacteria, which inoculate the infant during birth. Infants born through Cesarean section miss out on this colonization; they have lower numbers of the beneficial bifidobacteria and are more often colonized with the harmful bacteria C. difficile because they acquire bacteria from the hospital environment instead of from the mother.[3]

After birth, breastfed infants receive further advantage with improved gut bacteria as compared to exclusively formula-fed infants.[3] Another hindrance to the development of beneficial gut bacteria is antibiotic treatment during infancy, which is associated with decreased numbers of bifidobacteria. The establishment of gut flora is a progressive process, with increasing diversity important for overall health.[4] By age three, the major functions of the gut microbiota are established: nutrient absorption,immune stimulation, and protection against pathogens.

Throughout childhood, gut flora composition continues to develop until it reaches stability at the end of adolescence. In healthy adults, a diverse and stable gut flora (the GPS) will persist, contributing to digestive health as well as total body health. With age, however, modifications are seen in the gut microbial balance. Most notably, a decrease in beneficial bifidobacteria and an increase in potentially pathogenic bacteria occurs.[5]

There are a number of ways the gut flora, or GPS, can become imbalanced with decreased friendly bacteria and increased harmful bacteria. In the next chapter, learn about what factors contribute to gut imbalance, also known as dysbiosis. From poor diet and stress to certain medications, and yes, old age, the Gut Protection System faces many challenges along the way.

# The Human Microbiome Project

The human microbiome refers to the community of micro-organisms that populate the human body. The Human Microbiome Project was initiated by the National Institutes of Health (NIH) with the aim of characterizing the microbial communities found in and on different areas of the human body and associating changes in the microbiome with human health and disease. The $157 million project was launched in 2008 as part of the NIH Common Fund's Roadmap for Medical Research, and will involve increasingly complicated studies that aim to explain the role of the human microbiome in human health.

The advancement of technology involving DNA sequencing of microbes now allows for greater investigation of the human microbiome, and has changed the field of microbiology. With the new technology, a far greater understanding of microbial diversity is available. The Human Microbiome Project has set the following goals:

✓ Determining whether individuals share a common core human microbiome;

✓ Understanding changes in the human microbiome and to associate those changes to human health and disease; and

✓ Developing the new technological tools needed to support these goals.

# CHAPTER TWO

# GPS — What Can Go Wrong?

A careful balance of gut bacteria is what allows the Gut Protection System to function optimally. Though this balance is not completely understood, as science in this area is rapidly evolving, a balanced gut flora is generally accepted as a higher presence of good bacteria—like lactobacilli and bifidobacteria (the L's and the B's)—along with a low presence of potentially pathogenic bacteria—like clostridia or E. coli. A disruption in the balance of gut bacteria is known as dysbiosis, and can lead to health consequences in the digestive tract and in other areas of the body seemingly unrelated to the gut. Many factors can lead to the development of dysbiosis.

## Age

As mentioned in the previous chapter, age is a major contributor to gut imbalance. Levels of bifidobacteria and lactobacillus decrease with age, and so does bacterial diversity. Levels of potential pathogens increase, creating dysbiosis which may have detrimental effects on health.[6] With age often comes a decline in intestinal motility, or the ability of the intestines to move food through the digestive tract. This may result in constipation, a major problem in older adults. When food remains in the digestive tract for extended periods of time, as with constipation, bacterial protein fermentation occurs, creating a putrefactive environment due to the release of harmful bacterial metabolites, or by-products.[7] This is characteristic of dysbiosis.

## Diet

The Standard American Diet (SAD, an apt acronym) is high in sugar, animal protein, bad fats and artificial additives, and low in nutrients, fiber, lean proteins and good fats. The SAD diet contributes to an imbalanced GPS.

Potential pathogens thrive on the SAD diet while beneficial bacteria are at a disadvantage. A diet naturally high in fresh fruits and vegetables, whole grains, healthy fats and lean proteins best supports a healthy gut balance.

Beneficial bacteria, or probiotics, feed mostly on dietary fibers, prebiotic fibers and non-absorbed carbohydrates.[8] Prebiotic fibers are typically soluble fibers that act as food for beneficial bacteria while simultaneously reducing levels of harmful bacteria. Prebiotic fibers are found in chicory root, Jerusalem artichoke, dandelion greens, garlic, leeks, onions, asparagus, and in supplements of fructooligosaccharides (FOS) and acacia fiber.

In the past, fermented foods were a regular part of the diet because fermentation was a way to preserve food. Today, fermented foods are not as common, and in the case of yogurt, may not even contain live probiotics due to pasteurization. Consuming these foods might help balance the GPS, but it might not be enough.

A diet high in animal protein can contribute to unfavorable conditions in the gut due to the production of certain bacterial enzymes such as beta-glucuronidase, azoreductase and nitroreductase, which increase the release of toxins, including carcinogens, in the gut.[9] Further, with a high-protein diet, proteins may not be fully digested by the time they reach the colon where they can be fermented by gut bacteria that produce harmful metabolites.[10] A high-fiber diet is able to avoid this toxin buildup due to fiber's ability to absorb toxins and move intestinal contents through the digestive tract at an optimal pace.[11]

## Stress

The negative effects of stress involve the entire body, including the gut. Stress has become the norm in today's world. Stress can cause considerable changes to the gut microflora. Under stressful conditions, beneficial bacteria like lactobacilli and bifidobacteria decrease, and potentially pathogenic bacteria increase.[10]

Dysbiosis is not the only effect on the gut resulting from stress. Levels of the protective immunoglobulin secretory IgA (sIgA) are also reduced during stress. sIgA plays an important role in protecting the mucosal lining of the

9

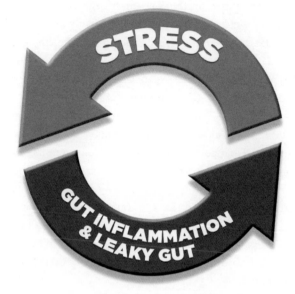

digestive tract by helping to protect against mucosal penetration by bacteria.[12] Further, stress increases gut inflammation and intestinal permeability, also known as leaky gut.[13] Thus begins a vicious cycle of gut dysfunction induced by stress, which, in turn, induces more stress, and the cycle continues. Stress reduction should always be a part of healing, for stress interferes with many physiological processes.

## Antibiotics

Antibiotics are the most common cause of imbalance in the GPS.[14] By definition the term *antibiotic* means, "against life." By contrast, *probiotic* means, "for life." Antibiotics work by killing the bacteria they encounter—both the good and the bad. This reduction of good gut bacteria creates a favorable environment for the bad bacteria to proliferate after antibiotic treatment. The result is an imbalanced GPS, and often, antibiotic-associated diarrhea (AAD).[15]

One of the most dangerous bacterial causes of AAD is *Clostridium difficile*, commonly called *C. diff*. *C. diff* is a normal inhabitant of the gut flora, and is kept in check by the friendly bacteria of the GPS. Antibiotic treatment weakens the protection of the GPS, however, allowing *C. diff* to flourish and release toxins that damage the intestinal lining, resulting in diarrhea.[16]

While antibiotic use is the trigger for *C.diff* infection, antibiotics are also the current treatment. This seeming paradox explains why *C.diff* infection has a high rate of recurrence. It is yet another vicious cycle.

Probiotics have been found effective for the prevention of antibiotic-associated diarrhea (AAD),[17] for the treatment of *C.difficile*-associated diarrhea, as well as for prevention of recurrent *C.diff* infections.[18] Probiotics help replenish the beneficial bacteria that are lost with antibiotic use, thus protecting against the proliferation of harmful pathogens.

Another potentially harmful organism found at low amounts in a healthy gut is the yeast Candida, most commonly *Candida albicans*. Candida presents a particularly difficult problem during antibiotic treatment because the yeast is not killed by antibiotics, which only kill bacteria. During antibiotic treatment when much of the gut bacteria is killed off, Candida is able to multiply without hindrance by the normal gut bacteria of the GPS. The resulting Candida overgrowth produces a toxic environment in the gut that is associated with symptoms like fatigue, brain fog, mood disorders, carb cravings, and more.

Parasites can also flourish when the GPS is out of balance. Parasites range from microscopic protozoa to worms reaching a length many feet long. When not kept under control by the GPS, parasites multiply and can interfere with proper immune function, consume nutrients meant to be absorbed and used by the body, and even migrate to other areas of the body. A study by Dr. Omar Amin found that one-third of the U.S. population has intestinal parasites.[19]

Antibiotics have greatly advanced modern medicine, no doubt, but the problem lies in their overuse. With repeated exposure to antibiotics, bacteria can become resistant to the antibiotics. Antibiotic resistance is an increasing problem, especially in hospitals. Many bacteria are developing antibiotic resistance, but the creation of new antibiotics to combat these so-called superbugs is not keeping pace with the rising number of antibiotic-resistant infections.[20,21]

One factor contributing to antibiotic resistance is the overprescription, and inappropriate prescription, of antibiotics. For example, many people are given antibiotics for the common cold, which is actually caused by a virus not killed by antibiotics. Other conditions treated unnecessarily with antibiotics include asthma, flu, cough, or ear infection.

## Acid-Suppressing Drugs

Another offender when it comes to interference with the GPS is acid-suppressing drugs. These include both antacids, like Tums, and acid-blockers or proton-pump inhibitors (PPIs), like Prilosec. We have been forced upon the idea that stomach acid is harmful, eating away at our stomach and esophagus, giving us acid indigestion and ulcers. This idea has been very profitable for the pharmaceutical industry because these drugs do ease symptoms of pain, like heartburn. But these medications are simply a band-aid solution to a deeper problem that involves more than over-production of stomach acid.

Stomach acid, also called gastric acid or hydrochloric acid (HCl), is a key component of a healthy digestive system. Stomach acid helps to break down proteins so that they are easier to digest by the digestive enzymes secreted in the GI tract. If stomach acid is too low, as opposed to too high—which is commonly the case—food is not properly broken down and can cause symptoms of heartburn, or, as the term clearly explains, *indigestion*.

Stomach acid also has another essential responsibility—to maintain an acidic environment in the stomach so that potential pathogens ingested with food, drink, or even air, can be killed as they pass through. When stomach acid is low, as occurs with acid-suppressing medications, pathogens can pass through the stomach into the intestines unhindered where they proliferate and can cause an infection.

Proton-pump inhibitors like Prilosec are not recommended for long-term use (read the label), however many people remain on these drugs for years at a time. Long-term use of PPIs alters the gut microflora,[22] producing side effects including abdominal pain, bloating, gas, constipation and diarrhea.[23] Further, long-term PPI use has been associated with increased risk of *C. difficile*-associated disease, development of esophageal candidiasis (Candida overgrowth in the esophagus), increased pneumonia infections, and even bone fracture in osteoporosis.[24,25,26,27]

Low stomach acid, or hypochlorhydria, is more common than most people realize. According to Dr. Jonathan Wright, M.D., author of *Why Stomach Acid is Good for You*, "When we actually measure stomach acid output under careful, research-verified conditions, the overwhelming majority of heartburn sufferers is found to have too little acid production. Even in severe cases diagnosed as GERD (gastroesophageal reflux disease), actual testing also shows hypochlorhydria in over 90 percent of cases."[28]

There is mounting evidence that suppression of stomach acid with medications like PPIs alters the gut flora, putting the GPS at a disadvantage. This points out the importance of getting to the core causes underlying conditions like heartburn, acid reflux and indigestion, before using medications that may do more harm in the long run.

## Environmental Toxins

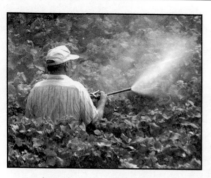

Over 80,000 chemicals have been introduced since the beginning of the 20th century with the onset of the Industrial Revolution. Of these many thousands of toxins, very few have been tested adequately for safety. From heavy metals and pesticides to artificial food ingredients and chemicals in beauty products, we are swimming in a toxic soup. In fact, the Environmental Working Group tested umbilical cord blood from 10 babies born in 2004, revealing a total of 287 different chemicals present in the group.[29] Toxins included pesticides, consumer product ingredients, and wastes from burning coal, gasoline, and garbage. Indeed, we are even born toxic.

Environmental toxins have been found to interfere with many of the body's processes. Many health conditions are triggered or worsened by toxins, and certain toxins have a negative impact on gut health, specifically. Heavy metals are particularly destructive to gut bacteria, creating dysbiosis in the gut.[30]

The GPS plays a major role in detoxification. Gut bacteria help to produce enzymes that work to break down and neutralize toxins in the gut so they can be carried out with bowel elimination.[31] Without a well-functioning GPS, toxins can be absorbed into the body, possibly overburdening the liver, the body's main organ of detoxification. The GPS works to help lower the body burden of toxins on the liver.

# CHAPTER THREE

# Getting Your GPS Back on Track with Probiotics

Good bacteria have been a part of the diet for thousands of years, largely in the form of fermented foods. One particular beneficial bacteria—bifidobacteria—was isolated from breast-fed newborns in 1899. This bacteria was then used to treat infants with diarrhea. The presence of this bacteria was, and still is, associated with good health.

In 1906 Elie Metchnikoff proposed the concept of the probiotic "Bulgarian bacillus," now known as *Lactobacillus bulgaricus*. Elie Metchnikoff is commonly referred to as the "Grandfather of Probiotics." His research and collaboration led to the modern interest in the ability of intestinal bacteria to benefit human health. He observed the long life spans of Bulgarians and attributed this to the fermented milk they drank. From this milk he isolated the *Lactobacillus* bacteria, and proposed that he could introduce this bacteria to the gut, producing a beneficial modification of the gut flora. Metchnikoff's research pointed out the adverse effects of "autointoxication"— the production of toxic gut bacterial metabolites that reached the bloodstream, resulting in poor health. Though the idea of autointoxication was not completely accepted for some time, recent research is validating this idea, illustrating the harmful effects of an imbalanced GPS on other areas of the body seemingly unrelated to the gut.

Today, probiotic research has greatly advanced. Probiotics are known to produce vitamins and enzymes, and enhance nutrient absorption necessary to health; they are in close communication with the immune system—80 percent of which resides in the gut—and help to balance immune response; and they help promote a healthy balance of bacteria in the gut, which protects against harmful bacteria and other pathogens.

# What Are Probiotics?

The World Health Organization and the Food and Agriculture Organization of the United Nations have offered the definition of "probiotics":[32]

*Probiotics are live microorganisms which when administered in adequate amounts confer a health benefit on the host.*

The host is you. This means that in order to truly be considered a probiotic, the organism(s) must be live when consumed, administered in the right amount, and must provide a health benefit to those who consume it.

Research on probiotics has increased dramatically over the past few decades. It is now recognized that individual probiotic strains have unique qualities. One strain may have specific immune-boosting properties, while another strain may have stronger ability to resist pathogens in the gut. For these reasons, and because of the wide diversity of bacteria that exists in the gut, a multi-strain probiotic formula more resembles that diversity, and may be more beneficial.[33]

Probiotics can be obtained through the diet by eating yogurt, kefir, and certain other fermented foods, but these products typically do not contain enough probiotic cultures to be of benefit. In fact, yogurt must be pasteurized, which involves high heat, so if probiotics are not re-added after pasteurization, the yogurt will not contain any beneficial bacteria.

Recently, many new probiotic products have appeared on store shelves, in supplements, foods, beverages, and even in gum. With all the variety, it can

# Your Gut Protection System

Have you heard that 80 percent of your immune system is found in the gut? That means the gut is the body's primary defense—think of the trillions of bacteria in the gut as your army. This army is what I call your GPS—your very own Gut Protection System—and it is the secret to good health. Let's look at how this process works using the example of a virus. Your friendly bacteria will fight off that virus on three different levels.

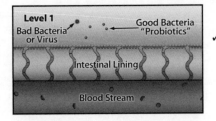

✓ **On Level 1**, while the virus is still in your intestinal tract, the good bacteria will surround and neutralize it.

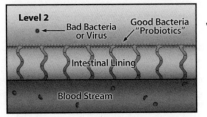

✓ **On Level 2**, the good bacteria will form a barrier along your intestinal lining and prevent the virus from passing through the intestinal lining and into the bloodstream.

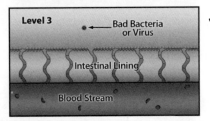

✓ **On Level 3**, if the virus even makes it that far, the friendly bacteria actually communicate with the immune system to produce substances that neutralize the virus before it causes damage.

What happens if these three levels are not working correctly? In Level 1, you'll get a build up of pathogenic bacteria that can make you sick. In Level 2, your intestinal lining barrier gets porous and lets in bad bacteria, toxins and parasites into the bloodstream. And in Level 3, the immune system will not be properly triggered to produce the substances that neutralize pathogens throughout the body.

be difficult to determine which products are high-quality. To be considered a "probiotic," the bacteria must go through a range of testing to ensure:[34]

✓ Identity: verified identification of species and strain.

✓ Safety: recognized as safe for human consumption.

✓ Stomach acid and bile resistance: ability to resist stomach acid and bile.

✓ Intestinal cell adhesion: ability to adhere to intestinal cells.

✓ Pathogen inhibition: ability to inhibit pathogenic bacteria by producing antimicrobial compounds, creating a protective barrier, and/or stimulating the immune system.

✓ Survival through the gastrointestinal tract: acid and bile resistance conferring the ability to pass through the GI tract in a viable state.

✓ Positive effect on the gut environment: produce favorable change in the gut.

✓ Health benefits: ability to improve gut function, and/or function of another area of health.

# CHAPTER FOUR

# The Gut Connection to Overall Health

As a nation, we've got serious digestion and elimination problems. One in five Americans, or as many as 20 percent of the adult population, experience symptoms of irritable bowel syndrome (IBS), one of the most commonly diagnosed health disorders. Because IBS is characterized by abdominal bloating, gas, cramping, diarrhea, and abdominal pain, it creates a number of digestive problems. Further, over four million Americans have frequent constipation requiring a doctor's visit. That is likely an underestimation, however, taking into account the many people who treat their constipation with over-the-counter laxatives, never visiting a doctor. Add to that the more than 60 million Americans who have heartburn at least once a month and the 15 million who experience symptoms daily—a more serious condition known as gastroesophageal reflux disease, or GERD—and we've got problems.

In addition to the many gastrointestinal conditions affecting Americans today, we are faced with an epidemic of cardiovascular disease, mood disorders like anxiety and depression, autoimmune conditions like type 1 diabetes and multiple sclerosis, and allergic conditions like asthma and eczema. You might think that these conditions have nothing to do with the gut, but you're wrong. Though the digestive system seems to be self-contained, the gut is the root and core of our overall health. In the gut, food is broken down into nutrients our body absorbs and uses for every function of the body. The gut is our first line of defense against pathogens and infections. The gut protects us against environmental toxins that can leak into the bloodstream. The gut is home to 80 percent of our immune system. I'm here to help you connect the dots between gut health and the health of the rest of your body.

The current study of the gut microflora and the use of probiotics to help treat and prevent GI conditions like irritable bowel syndrome and antibiotic-associated diarrhea, is one of the most exciting developments of science.

But even more exciting is the science currently underway that is finding the gut connection to many different areas of health throughout the whole body. Studies have shown that probiotics can help improve immunity and contribute to everything from dental health to mental health, women's health, metabolic health and more. For additional information on probiotic studies, visit www.probiotic-research.com

## PROBIOTICS AND GUT HEALTH CONDITIONS

### Irritable Bowel Syndrome

Irritable bowel syndrome (IBS) is not only one of the most common digestive complaints, it's also one of the most common overall health disorders diagnosed by doctors. IBS is characterized by an alteration in bowel habit—either predominantly constipation, predominantly diarrhea, or, most commonly, an alternation between the two. Symptoms of IBS include abdominal pain, bloating, discomfort, and the feeling of incomplete bowel elimination.

Though IBS is largely thought of as a functional bowel disorder with no apparent physical changes, recent research is uncovering an imbalance in the gut microflora—the GPS—as an underlying feature of IBS. Studies have found that people with IBS have a relative reduction in lactobacilli and bifidobacteria (the L's and the B's) and increases in other potentially pathogenic bacteria.[35] These changes in gut bacteria affect the gut mucosal barrier (the protective lining of the digestive tract) and immune response, both of which contribute to the symptoms of IBS.[36]

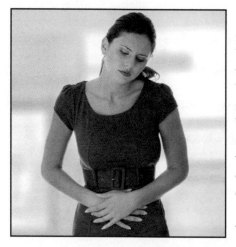

One particular form of dysbiosis is known as small intestinal bacterial overgrowth (SIBO), which involves an overgrowth of bacteria at the end of the small intestine more resembling the bacteria of the colon. In one study, 78 percent of IBS patients were found to have SIBO, and eradication of the bacterial overgrowth was able to eliminate IBS in 48 percent of those people with SIBO and IBS.[37]

The major role that the Gut Protection System plays in IBS has led to many studies investigating the use of probiotics to alleviate IBS symptoms. IBS is a difficult condition to treat, requiring a multi-pronged approach.[35] In one study, a multi-strain probiotic containing *Lactobacillus acidophilus*, *Bifidobacterium lactis* and *Bifidobacterium bifidum* was administered for eight weeks to patients with IBS. Compared to placebo, a significantly greater improvement in symptom severity and in quality of life was observed.[38] Similar results are found for a variety of probiotics strains, though care should be taken when selecting probiotics, for not all strains are found to be of benefit for IBS.

## Antibiotic-Associated Diarrhea

Antibiotic-associated diarrhea is a common side effect of antibiotic treatment, especially in a hospital setting. Antibiotics work by killing bacteria—both good and bad. The result can be antibiotic-associated diarrhea, sometimes caused by the potential pathogen *Clostridium difficile* (also known as *C.diff*). When the beneficial bacteria are disrupted with antibiotics, the gut becomes imbalanced, causing digestive symptoms and leaving the gut vulnerable to attack by potential pathogens. The GPS gets thrown off track.

One study, commissioned by the Association for Professionals in Infection Control and Epidemiology, found that on any given day over 7,000 hospitalized patients are infected with *C.difficile* and about 300 of those people will end up dying from the infection.[39]

The use of probiotics to help rebuild the GPS during and after antibiotic treatment can help to thwart the digestive disturbance of *C.diff* by assisting with the reestablishment of the intestinal microflora, enhancing immune response, and by inhibiting pathogens and their toxins. A variety of probiotics have been found effective for antibiotic-associated diarrhea (AAD) and *C. difficile*-associated diarrhea (CDAD).[40]

## Infectious Diarrhea and Traveler's Diarrhea

Infectious diarrhea involves diarrhea caused by a pathogen, usually a virus, but sometimes a bacteria or parasite. Most of the time the specific organism is not tested for, and the diarrhea is allowed to run its course with appropriate rehydration therapy. Traveler's diarrhea involves an intestinal infection acquired during travel to another country. Consuming contaminated food or drink, such as tap water, ice, non-pasteurized milk, or raw fruits and vegetables, puts travelers at risk for developing traveler's diarrhea, especially in areas of high incidence like northern Africa, Latin America, the Middle East and Southeast Asia.[41]

Because diarrhea involves a major disruption to the intestinal tract, probiotics have been investigated as treatment and prevention of both infectious and traveler's diarrhea. One meta-analysis of 12 studies found probiotics to be effective in the prevention of traveler's diarrhea.[41] Several probiotics were found to be effective — *S. boulardii*, a mixture of *L. acidophilus* and *B. bifidum*, and a multi-strain probiotic formula. All probiotics prevented diarrhea significantly more than placebo. In a Cochrane Systematic Review of 23 studies of probiotics for the treatment of infectious diarrhea, probiotics were found to be a useful addition to rehydration therapy in both adults and children.[42] By reinforcing the gut with probiotics, the GPS can function optimally to defend against potential pathogens.

## Constipation

Constipation is one of the most common digestive conditions, with more than 4 million Americans reporting frequent bouts of constipation. This estimate is likely low, since many people do not seek medical consultation for constipation, instead treating it with over-the-counter medication, or not treating it at all. Constipation is defined by traditional medicine as fewer than three bowel movements per week. Many natural health practitioners define constipation as fewer than one bowel movement per day, however.

Probiotics can be helpful for people with constipation for a few reasons. First, studies have found a difference in the intestinal microflora between healthy individuals and those with constipation (constipated people have higher amounts of potentially pathogenic clostridia bacteria, for example).[43] Second, a number of studies have found probiotics to help increase colonic transit time, which improves constipation.[44] And last, probiotics help to reduce the pH of the colon, due to the production of beneficial short chain fatty acids and lactic acid. Lower pH enhances peristalsis of the colon,[45] which is the contraction of the colon that propels its contents through the GI tract.

## Upper GI Conditions

Upper GI conditions involve the upper GI tract—the esophagus and stomach—and include heartburn and GERD (gastroesophageal reflux

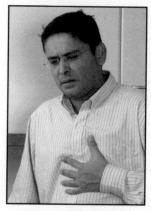

disease, also known as acid reflux), esophagitis, Barrett's esophagus, gastritis and peptic ulcers. These conditions are often treated with acid-suppressing medications. As mentioned in Chapter Two, the long-term use of acid-blocking medications, specifically proton-pump inhibitors (PPIs), is associated with a range of adverse effects.

One of the harmful effects of suppressing stomach acid is the alteration of the gut microbiota. Because these medications decrease stomach acid, harmful bacteria can pass through the stomach without hindrance, and proliferate in the intestines where they create an imbalance in the GPS, or dysbiosis. Use of PPI medications is associated with the development of small intestinal bacterial overgrowth (SIBO) together with irritable bowel syndrome (IBS), suggesting that PPIs may be at the root cause of some cases of IBS.[23]

Because gut imbalance can result from medications used to treat upper GI conditions, use of probiotics may be helpful. In fact, probiotics have been found to improve treatment of *Helicobacter pylori* (H. pylori) infection, a bacteria that causes gastritis, peptic ulcer and stomach cancer. Adding probiotics to standard therapy for H. pylori, which includes antibiotics and PPIs, has been found to improve the treatment.[46]

## OTHER BENEFITS OF PROBIOTICS – THE GUT CONNECTION

The digestive health benefits of probiotics are obvious—beneficial gut bacteria help bring about digestive balance. It makes sense to fortify your GPS with an army that's on your side. But probiotics also have beneficial effects for areas of the body seemingly unrelated to the gut. This is possible due to the connection of the gut to all other areas of the body. With 80 percent of your immune system in your gut, more nerve cells in your gut than in your brain, and a direct blood supply from the gut to the rest of the body, it's little surprise that probiotics promote more than just digestive health.

### Immunity

The gut microflora serves as the first line of defense for the immune system by creating a protective barrier along the intestinal lining. This helps keep potential pathogens from reaching the gut lining, and protects against increased intestinal permeability, or leaky gut.[47] If the GPS is out of balance, this defense barrier is compromised, and so is immunity. Because 80 percent of the immune system resides in the gut, probiotics can have a notable effect on immune health.

**The immune system has two main functions:**

- To respond to potential pathogens by inhibiting and destroying them, and to remember each one so that the next time they are encountered a more extensive response can be mounted against them; and
- To *not* mount an attack against that which does not pose a threat to the body, i.e. food, other cells of the body, or harmless ingested particles.

Basically, a balanced immune response needs to occur. In a healthy person, the immune system simultaneously responds to invaders while tolerating harmless particles passing through. An example of an out-of-balanced immune response would be low immune response to viral illnesses like cold and flu, or, alternately, an over-response of the immune system as seen with autoimmunity, which involves the immune system mistaking the body's own cells as invaders, and destroying those cells. Autoimmune conditions include inflammatory bowel disease, type 1 diabetes and multiple sclerosis.

A balanced immune response is ideal. Probiotics are particularly helpful to the immune system because they help to balance immune response. They help to educate the immune system so it responds appropriately. For example, probiotics have been found to reduce incidence of cold and flu, relieve symptoms, and reduce the use of antibiotics for cold and flu episodes in children.[48] Further, an alteration of the gut microbiota is thought to play a major role in the development of autoimmune conditions.[49]

### Allergies

Allergies are another example of imbalanced immune response. With allergies, whether inhaled allergies like rhinitis and asthma; food allergies involving ingested allergens; or atopic dermatitis, a form of allergic response manifested in the skin, the immune system overreacts in response to normal antigens like food.

The increasing incidence of allergic diseases in developed countries has been linked to the decreased exposure to environmental microbes, due to decreased

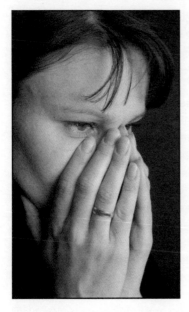

family size, improved hygiene, vaccination, antibiotics, and the consumption of sterile foods.[50] This is known as the Hygiene Hypothesis.

Children who grow up in less sterile environments, who are raised on farms, who attend daycare and thus experience more infections during infancy and early childhood, or who are supplemented with the probiotic *Lactobacillus ruminus* are less likely to develop allergies and allergic asthma later in life.[51] This is largely because the microbes to which these children are exposed serve to educate their immune systems, essentially priming the immune system to respond appropriately.

For obvious reasons, it is not possible to revert back to less hygienic living, so alternatives to microbial exposure must be found. Probiotics are safe alternatives for providing the microbial exposure missing from Western cultures.[50] In one study in infants with eczema, feeding of hydrolyzed infant formula supplemented with *Bifidobacterium lactis* or *Lactobacillus rhamnosus* was found to reduce recovery time from six months to two months.[52] Probiotics have also been found to prevent the development of eczema. Pregnant mothers with allergic disease were given *Lactobacillus rhamnosus* or placebo from 2 to 4 weeks before their delivery due date; after birth, the infants were also given the probiotics for six months. After four years, 46 percent of the placebo group had developed eczema compared to only 26 percent of the probiotic group.[53]

**Probiotics may influence allergy by protecting the GPS in the following ways:** [50]

- Protection of mucosal barrier function
- Breakdown of food allergens
- Improvement of gut microbial balance
- Reduction of inflammation
- Direct immune modulation

After the colon, the region most concentrated with bacteria is the vagina. In healthy women, lactobacilli bacteria are prevalent. Lactobacilli produce lactic acid and hydrogen peroxide, which promote a more acidic vaginal pH. This lower pH protects against bacterial pathogens which require a higher pH to thrive. Many factors can alter the vaginal microflora, however, such as hormone changes, hygiene practices, medications (like birth control pills) and even the gut bacteria.

In four studies using different combinations of *Lactobacillus* probiotics, bacterial vaginosis was alleviated compared to placebo or to antibiotic treatment.[33] The species found most beneficial were *L. rhamnosus*, *L. reuteri*, *L. salivarius*, *L. plantarum*, *L acdidophilus* and *L. casei*. Though some studies administered probiotics vaginally, orally administered probiotics have been found to colonize the vagina.[54]

Yeast infections, usually caused by the yeast *Candida albicans*, are particularly common in women, and often occur following antibiotic treatment. This is because yeast are not killed by antibiotics, and are able to proliferate uninhibited. Taking probiotics during and after antibiotic treatment can help to mitigate this problem. Daily support with probiotics has been found to reduce recurrent yeast infections.[55] Probiotics have also been found to prevent recurrent urinary tract infections in women in a number of clinical studies. The most effective strains were *L. rhamnosus*, *L. reuteri*, *L. casei* and *L.crispatus*.[56]

## Arthritis

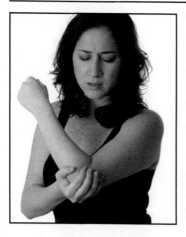

Though arthritis seems about as far from the gut as you can get, there is a clear gut connection to the condition. In fact, in one study, 56 percent of patients with inflammatory arthritis were found to have either gut dysbiosis or genitourinary dysbiosis (vaginal flora imbalance).[57]

The gut connection to arthritis was nicely illustrated in an interesting study that looked at the fecal bacterial balance of people with rheumatoid arthritis after eating a vegetarian diet for 13 months. The study found that patients on the diet increased the amount of beneficial bacteria in the colon, which was associated with an improvement in their arthritis.[58]

In patients with inflammatory bowel disease (IBD), a multi-strain probiotic formula was found to improve arthritis pain, a common affliction in IBD.[59] In another study, a single strain probiotic was found to improve pain scores in people with rheumatoid arthritis.[60] Clearly, there is a gut-connection to arthritis.

## Cardiovascular Disease

Cardiovascular disease is the number one cause of death in the U.S. The connection between gut health and cardiovascular health may seem obscure, but it's not. One interesting study looked at intestinal function in people with chronic heart failure. The study found that intestinal permeability, or leaky gut, in addition to bacterial overgrowth, contributed to the inflammation that is found in chronic heart failure.[61]

Another study found that people who ate a high-fat meal had higher levels of bacterial toxins (lipopolysaccharides, or LPS) in their blood than did people who ate a low-fat meal.[62] Increased amounts of LPS in the bloodstream contribute to the development of atherosclerosis. LPS is produced by potentially pathogenic bacteria (gram negative) and enters the bloodstream primarily by way of a leaky gut. This is an important gut-heart connection that is being studied further.

## Diabetes

Similar to cardiovascular disease, dysbiosis may also play a role in the development of type 2 diabetes. One study found that increased levels of the bacterial toxin lipopolysaccharide (LPS) in the blood triggered insulin resistance and obesity.[63] The study also found that a high-fat diet triggered the increase of LPS in association with a change in gut bacteria. In another study, intestinal bacteria in people with diabetes was found to be different from that of healthy people.[64] As with cardiovascular disease, this is an exciting area of research currently under way.

## Obesity

Gut bacteria have also been found to play a role in obesity. In both humans and mice, differences were found in the gut bacteria of obese and lean individuals.[65]

It is thought that the bacteria associated with obese individuals, called the 'obese microbiota,' were involved in harvesting more calories from food that passed through the intestines, thus resulting in weight gain.

Another study highlighting the connection between the GPS and obesity involved pregnant women. Those women who were given probiotic supplements containing lactobacilli and bifidobacteria during their entire pregnancy were found to have the lowest levels of abdominal obesity one year after childbirth.[66]

## Gut-Brain Connection

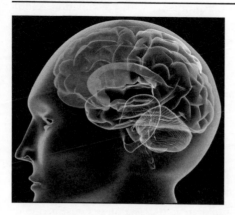

The gut-brain connection occurs in two directions—from the brain to the gut, and from the gut to the brain. When you get a "gut feeling" or feel "butterflies" in your stomach, the brain is sending a message to the gut. The digestive tract is sensitive to emotions. Just as an anxious brain can affect your gut, a distressed gut can affect the brain.

The gut houses the enteric nervous system, a part of the peripheral nervous system that is made up of 100 million neurons connecting the gut to the brain. When the gut is in a state of dysbiosis, the GPS is off track. The result is inflammation in the gut. This gut inflammation triggers the immune system to respond in a chain reaction that produces yet more inflammation in the form of inflammatory cytokines. Inflammatory cytokines from peripheral areas of the body (like the gut) have been found to activate the brain and induce behaviors of anxiety, depression and mood changes.[67]

A randomized, double-blind, placebo-controlled trial investigated the effects of a specific strain of *Lactobacillus casei* on emotional symptoms in people with chronic fatigue syndrome, a condition commonly associated with depression and anxiety. The probiotic was found to increase fecal concentrations of both lactobacilli and bifidobacteria, as well as decrease anxiety symptoms.[68] Results of this study support the gut-brain connection concept, illustrating the beneficial effects brought about by balancing the GPS.

# CHAPTER FIVE

# Success Stories

Let me tell you about my experience helping my dad. He is now 87 and for several years he has had chronic problems with constipation. Many of his doctors felt that as long as he had a movement once every two or three days he was OK. The doctors' recommendations included Dulcolax, Miralax, milk of magnesia, polyethylene glycol, magnesium citrate, as well as prescription medications. He was taking several of these at the same time. He was having problems so bad with compaction that he made several trips to the emergency room.

About a year ago, I had his caretaker give him your First Cleanse 2-week program then followed up with one capsule daily of the Ultimate Flora Senior 30 Billion probiotic at bedtime and the Daily Multi-Detox (no laxative in this) 2 capsules before bedtime. We discontinued all the other doctor-recommended products. He has not had even one problem with digestion or constipation in over a year! He has gained needed weight while eating less food. He got so much healthier that the regular home health nursing care that he had been receiving for six years was discontinued!

Thanks so much for your over-the-phone Personal Cleansing Coaches!

—Larry F, TN

I am on day five and can't believe how much better I feel!

—Nancy C

I love your Ultimate Flora Senior formula. I no longer need Nexium. Your product is fantastic! I've tried other prescription medications besides Nexium and they did not work. Your product has left me heartburn- and reflux-free!

—Trisha M, Naples, FL

For most of my adult years I was plagued by urinary tract infections (almost monthly). Until approximately 10 years ago my doctor treated me for these infections . . . but they always returned. I am a very healthy woman on no medication other than those to treat the infections, so I decided to research a natural product to fight these infections. I found ReNew Life Ultimate Flora Critical Care 50 Billion. I've been taking one capsule in the evening for over three years and have had no sign of the infections that I had for so many years. I believe Ultimate Flora rid my body of the unhealthy bacteria that caused these infections, so I'll be taking this product permanently.

—Jan B.

We recently purchased Ultimate Flora Critical Care 50 Billion. My 13-year-old son has been suffering with stomach pains for over a year since major surgery. He was on many pain killers and took ibuprofen during his recovery. He has been to a gastroenterologist, allergist, and a naturopathic practitioner. While some of his allergies had been diagnosed, he was still having pain after almost every meal, and some nights he couldn't sleep at all. He missed many many days of school. Since he started taking the Ultimate Flora Critical Care 50 Billion, it is like a miracle! He is able to eat without pain, and he even ate some Mexican food that we thought might trigger the problem again, but it didn't. We are so amazed and thankful! Your product is an answer to our many prayers!

—Renee, CA

I am 46 and have dealt with allergy symptoms for most of my adult life; at times the symptoms were so severe I couldn't carry on "normally." About 11 years ago I was diagnosed with asthma, which is just an allergic symptom in the lungs, and was prescribed inhalers, one being a steroid. I found, to my astonishment, that one time I needed to use eight puffs a day of the steroid inhaler for about a week, I got severe laryngitis. An overactive immune response (asthma) also ups mucous production and causes wheezing and tightness. So I was always coughing because my body wanted to get the mucous out.

I recently discovered that about 70 percent of the immune system resides in the gut and that an imbalance of bacteria can affect immune response. I then thought about the fact that over the years I had been on antibiotics many times and was not informed by any doctor that they not only kill the bad bacteria, but also the good. I decided to try Ultimate Flora and I am so glad I did. I cannot begin to tell you how great I feel. After I started the product, I immediately noticed an improvement in all my allergic symptoms, mostly the asthma. I have not had to use any inhalers for the past week, and I am looking forward to many more weeks with no inhalers. Research/knowledge gives one power and choices.

—Kathryn K

Thank you so much for your Ultimate Flora Critical Care 50 Billion. My 9-year-old son, Colin, has been struggling with diarrhea off and on for three years! It was so bad at Christmas time that he was dehydrated, weak, and vomiting. I was desperate when a good friend told me to give Colin DiarEase and Ultimate Flora, three per day, to start. Within 12 hours his diarrhea was gone, and now 10 days later, every day is still a good day for Colin! His energy is amazing and he is so happy to be better. We can never thank you enough!

—Colleen M

Here is my story of the wonderful results I have had using your ReNew Life Products recovering from a recent battle with C-diff and ulcerative colitis (UC).

My business brings me into contact with institutions known for a high incidence of C-diff among their residents or patients. Our clients include hospital groups, national ACLF chains and residential environments where patient have home health care. My history with colon challenges goes back to 2002 when I had my first bout with UC. This was a new experience for me, as at that time I was a healthy 51-year-old man with an active lifestyle. While I knew you then, I did not have but a passing contact with ReNew Life at that time, though I pursued a healthy lifestyle and diet as a result of this experience. I broke training several years later and again had a flare-up of UC in 2007 resulting in a second hospital stay and more strict diet and lifestyle changes.

I responded well to these changes and until May of 2010 I felt I had it pretty well under control. In May, I started again to have UC symptoms and immediately started back on the strictest dietary program and supplements thinking that I would have this under control in a week or so. Unbeknownst to me, C. diff had similar symptoms and would not be affected by my dietary and supplemental routine. UC suffers are also more prone to this type of infection due to their compromised colon terrain.

Three weeks and a loss of 35 pounds later, I asked to be admitted due to chronic diarrhea and dehydration. Within a few hours of being admitted to the hospital, I was diagnosed with C. diff and isolated. They started me on a massive antibiotic regimen and gave me a probiotic capsule three times a day. I wish I was working with you then as I know my recovery would have been more rapid in conjunction with allopathic treatment.

A friend who manages the vitamin department at a large health food store advised me of the Ultimate Flora Super Critical 200 Billion, and I started taking that once a day while still in the hospital and on antibiotics. (My doctor was advised and approved.) I had no appetite and was continuing to lose weight. When I was discharged after 10 days, I went home feeling as sick as I ever have in my life. I had no energy or desire to eat and felt like my life was slowly slipping away. Though I was already on the ReNew Life program, I was not gaining any ground. After meeting with Tracy [of ReNew Life] in mid July, a ReNew Life protocol was designed for me. Within a few days of starting the program I noticed a positive change in the constitution of my bowel movements, and the bloating in my gut was beginning to subside.

Six weeks later and I am continuing to gain weight and my energy is returning steadily. I am back at work and feeling productive again. I know that the program designed for me was critical to my healing and I can state without doubt that I will continue to consult with ReNew Life and stay on my specific carbohydrate diet. If not for your help, I feel that my recovery would have been greatly inhibited. My GI doctor is impressed with my continued improvement and is considering how it may have a positive impact on his other patients.

As of today, I know I am on the right path and have the tools at my disposal to achieve the best health possible. With a good diet, the right supplements, and a healthy lifestyle, the possibilities are limitless for a long and productive life ahead of me. Thank you for all your help.

—Will S

In August 2008, I started to feel pains in my abdomen. After three days they became more localized and I suspected appendicitis and went to my doctor, who immediately sent me to the Emergency Room. My diagnosis was appendicitis with possible rupture, and the treatment was immediate appendectomy. The surgery was done laparoscopically, and later that afternoon I was already able to walk around my hospital ward. Twentyseven hours after admission I was able to go home. The next day I put in about half a day in the office, and on the third day after surgery I worked all day.

The fourth day was a big surprise. I had severe diarrhea and was so tired that I could hardly get out of bed. I assumed that I had overdone it and expected to be much better by the next day, but I was not much stronger and the diarrhea was worse. I made it to work feeling really bad and called my doctor, who asked me to come in for tests. My stool sample was processed very rapidly and they called to tell me that, as they had suspected, I had contracted something I'd never heard of called clostridium difficile, better known as c. difficile or C.Diff.

I returned to the surgeon's office and he prescribed the antibiotic vancomycin. Since he was the very man who had saved my life just the previous week, I did not question his advice or prescription, but immediately began the 10-day course of antibiotics. After only two days on the antibiotic I was much improved, and by the fourth day my diarrhea and tiredness were gone. I finished the antibiotics on the tenth day as prescribed.

I drove across the state of Florida from Fort Lauderdale to Tampa and during this nightmare drive all my symptoms returned. By then I had read more about C. Diff so I knew that many strains develop immunity to antibiotics—they literally go underground until the antibiotic is gone and then return with a vengeance.

Fortunately—by coincidence—the next day I had a business meeting with Brenda Watson. I looked rough when I got to her office and quickly shared my story. She knew a lot about C. Diff and together we developed a treatment strategy. She also arranged for another stool sample to be tested so we could establish the seriousness of my "infestation." The stool test results showed that I also had some other mysterious and potentially harmful bacteria, as well as yeast and very high inflammation markers.

My treatment would be very large doses of probiotics on the principle that these beneficial bacteria would literally crowd out the C. Diff bacteria. During the course of antibiotics, I had taken ReNew Life's Ultimate Flora Critical Care 50 Billion, which contains fifty billion bacteria per capsule—the highest dose of probiotics I could find.

After further study and a couple more days in which I felt slightly better, I stepped up my dose to about 1 trillion probiotic units per day—about 20 high-dose capsules. I also reported my relapse to my surgeon who told me that he would prescribe another antibiotic—Flagyl. However, in some studies in Europe, C. Diff had recurred in 80 percent of cases after five courses of antibiotics! I thanked him and said I would trust in probiotics and get back to him if I needed more antibiotics.

After another two weeks in which I made steady progress each day, I felt almost normal and gradually cut down my probiotic dose to about 400 billion units per day. Then, over a weekend, I forgot to take it and the diarrhea returned. So I got back on the probiotic wagon and gradually reduced my daily dose to about 100 billion units per day. My latest test results showed no C. Diff.

So, if you have C.Diff, you may have success with antibiotics, but if not, try a lot of probiotics and if my experience is anything to go by, you may well be able to overwhelm those nasty bacteria. Good luck. Either way, Brenda Watson's fantastic advice and ReNew Life's Ultimate Flora will help

—Roy B

For more information on ReNew Life products, visit www.renewlife.com

# Summary

As it turns out, "the road to perfect health" is paved with good intestines. Rapidly evolving research supports the critical role of the gut flora in maintaining digestive and overall health. From infancy, the protective gut flora acts as the body's "Gut Protection System," or GPS. In today's world, building and maintaining a healthy GPS is a challenge due to the overuse of antibiotics, acid-suppressing medications, poor diet and environmental toxin exposure. An imbalanced GPS is linked to common digestive conditions like irritable bowel syndrome (IBS), diarrhea and constipation, in addition to conditions involving many different areas of the body, like allergies, diabetes, obesity and anxiety.

The science behind the gut microflora is rapidly expanding and researchers are finding more applications for probiotics as science advances. Certain probiotic strains, mostly the lactobacilli and bifidobacteria, have been well-studied for digestive conditions like irritable bowel syndrome (IBS) and antibiotic-associated diarrhea (AAD). This research encourages the acceptance of probiotics by mainstream medicine, and is the incentive for further research of probiotics on conditions affecting other areas of the body.

Probiotics help maintain digestive balance in healthy people, and can help bring about gut balance in people with digestive upsets. Specific probiotic lactobacilli and bifidobacteria strains have been found to support immunity, protect against allergies, support women's vaginal health, reduce arthritic pain, and even reduce anxiety. The gut connection to overall health is clear— if you have a colon you should be taking probiotics!

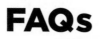

# FAQs

### How do probiotics work?

Probiotics are live microorganisms that provide a benefit to the host—that's you. When the Gut Protection System, or GPS becomes imbalanced (with too many harmful bacteria, and too little friendly bacteria), digestive upsets and poor health may result. Probiotics support intestinal balance by "crowding out" and inhibiting the harmful bacteria, protecting the intestinal lining, and by communicating with the immune system for reinforcement.

### Are probiotics safe?

The *Lactobacillus* and *Bifidobacterium* probiotic strains, as well as *S. boulardii*, have been well studied and characterized for safety. Make sure the probiotic you choose contains strains that have undergone safety studies.

### Can I consume probiotics from foods?

It is possible to obtain some probiotics by eating fermented foods like yogurt, kefir or sauerkraut, but it can be difficult to obtain enough probiotic cultures with these foods alone. Further, knowing what strains and how many cultures are present can be difficult with these foods. With yogurt, if the probiotics are not added after pasteurization, there will not be any probiotics present due to the high heat required during the pasteurization process.

### Are high-potency probiotics safe?

Probiotics are safe at high doses. In animals models, which are the standard for safety studies of high dosage, no lethal dose has been achievable. Multi-strain probiotics have been safely consumed at levels well over 900 billion per day in humans.

# How do I choose a probiotic supplement?

When shopping for an effective probiotic supplement, consumers should read labels carefully to ensure the following:

- **High Culture Count.** This refers to the total amount of bacteria per serving Look for a probiotic supplement with at least 15 billion cultures in a single capsule.

- **Number of Strains.** Your supplement should include at least 10 different strains of bacteria scientifically proven to benefit optimal health. Look for high amounts of *Bifidobacterium* to support the large intestine (colon) and *Lactobacillus* to support the small intestine and urogenital tract.

- **Delayed Release Capsules.** Delayed release capsules protect the probiotics from harsh stomach acid and deliver them directly to the intestines where they are needed and utilized by the body.

- **Potency & Stability Guarantee.** The potency, or amount of active cultures, should be guaranteed through the product expiration date under recommended storage conditions.

Other important things to look for:

- **Clearly Stated Information on Label.** Includes Supplement Facts, dosing information, and directions for use/storage. Many products have complicated dosing regimens or directions, and the suggested storage conditions vary based on probiotic form and stability.

- **Reputable Manufacturer.** Look for products manufactured by well-trusted companies who have a history of good clinical evidence and support for their products. Contact details such as a website or toll-free number should be featured prominently.

- **"Best Used By" Date and Batch or Lot Code.** The code printed on an individual container serves as a reference number for the plant to track production information.

## Do probiotics boost immunity?

Actually, probiotics work to balance immune response. They boost immune response, yet also offer anti-inflammatory properties that can quell an overactive immune system. This is why they have been found beneficial both for conditions involving poor immunity, like cold and flu, as well as conditions of overactive immunity like autoimmune conditions. Probiotics help educate the immune system so it responds appropriately.

## Are all probiotics equal?

No. Research shows that probiotics are strain specific, meaning that certain strains have distinctive properties that are not shared with other similar strains. Some strains have specific properties against certain pathogens, while others have particular anti-inflammatory properties. This is why a multi-strain formula is the best approach.

## Do specific probiotic strains benefit certain parts of the digestive tract differently than others?

*Lactobacillus* strains are most prevalent in the small intestine, and *Bifidobacteria* strains are most prevalent in the large intestine. For this reason, it is best to find a probiotic formula that contains a variety of the L's (for little intestine) and the B's (for big intestine).

# PROBIOTIC QUESTIONNAIRE

Discover the Best Probiotic for YOU!

How do you know you're getting the right probiotic for your health concern, age or particular situation? Let this handy guide clear up the confusion and help put you on The Road to Perfect Health!

**Q.** Are you a healthy adult aged 15 to 49 who wants to maintain a healthy balance of friendly gut bacteria? (See p.5)

**A.** Look for a high-count (15 billion CFU), multi-strain probiotic high in Bifidobacteria strains formulated for adults.

**Q.** Are you a healthy adult over the age of 50 who wants to maintain a healthy balance of friendly gut bacteria because levels of Bifidobacteria decline after age 50? (See p. 6)

**A.** Look for a high-count (30 billion CFU), multi-strain probiotic high in Bifidobacteria strains formulated specifically for seniors.

**Q.** Are you taking, or have recently completed, a course of antibiotics? Or do you have a particularly troublesome digestive tract? (See p. 10)

**A.** Look for a high-count (50 billion CFU), multi-strain probiotic high in Bifidobacteria strains formulated specifically for critical care.

**Q.** Are you a woman who is concerned about the balance of healthy vaginal bacteria and yeast, or want to support a healthy urinary tract? (See p. 25)

**A.** Look for a high-count (50 billion CFU), multi-strain probiotic high in Lactobacillus strains formulated specifically for vaginal health.

**Q.** Are you concerned about an acute phase of illness or stress and want to rebalance your digestive tract? (See p. 9)

**A.** Look for a maximum-count (200 billion CFU), multi-strain probiotic in powder form that also contains 2,000 mg of FOS, a prebiotic that helps to boost levels of healthy bacteria.

**Q.** Do you have acute lower intestinal/colon care needs—such as occasional irritable bowel, diarrhea, constipation or digestive discomfort—and would like to rebalance your gut bacteria? (See p. 19)

**A.** Look for a high-count (80 billion CFU), multi-strain probiotic that contains a wide range of Bifidobacteria strains formulated specifically for colon health.

**Q.** Do you want extra immune support for seasonal health conditions affecting the lungs and respiratory system especially in spring and winter? (See p. 22)

**A.** Look for a probiotic formula that contains 10 billion cultures of Saccharomyces Boulardii, as well as the ingredients EpiCor® and ResistAid™, that is specifically formulated for immune support.

**Q.** Do you travel often, or are you planning a trip and want to maintain digestive health while away? (See p. 20)

**A.** Look for a maximum-count (200 billion CFU), multi-strain probiotic in powder form that comes in convenient packets that can be carried with you when you're away.

**Q.** Do you have trouble swallowing pills but want to maintain a healthy balance of beneficial gut bacteria?

**A.** Look for a maximum-count (200 billion CFU), multi-strain probiotic in powder form that can be easily added to cold foods or liquid.

**Q.** Do you have upper GI concerns that involve the stomach or esophagus? (See p. 21)

**A.** Look for a maximum-count (200 billion), multi-strain probiotic in powder form that can be easily added to cold foods or liquid so that it comes into direct contact with the upper digestive lining.

# Resources

## Websites

Natural Center for Complimentary and Alternative Medicine. Probiotics.
www.nccam.nih.gov/health/probiotics/

National Digestive Diseases Information Clearninghouse.
www.digestive.niddk.nih.gov

International Foundation for Functional Gastrointestinal Disorders.
http://www.iffgd.org

International Scientific Association for Probiotics and Prebiotics.
www.isapp.net

Digestive Care Expert Brenda Watson
www.brendawatson.com

Comprehensive Library of Research on Probiotics
www.probiotic-research.com

## Books

Wright J and Lenard L, *Why Stomach Acid is Good for You.* M Evans and Co, Inc, 2001.

Floch MH and Kim AS, Eds., *Probiotics A Clinical Guide,* SLACK Inc., 2010.

Brenda Watson, C.N.C. *The Road to Perfect Health: Balance Your Gut, Heal Your Body.* ReNew Life Press (2010).

Brenda Watson, C.N.C. *Gut Solutions: Natural Solutions to Your Digestive Problems.* ReNew Life Press (2004).

Brenda Watson, C.N.C. *The H.O.P.E. Formula: The Ultimate Health Secret.* ReNew Life Press (2007).

Brenda Watson, C.N.C. *The Fiber35 Diet: Nature's Weight Loss Secret.* Free Press (2008).

Brenda Watson, C.N.C. *The Detox Strategy: Vibrant Health in 5 Easy Steps.* Free Press (2009).

## Products

ReNew Life Ultimate Flora Probiotics. www.renewlife.com www.ultimateflora.com
Fiber35 Diet. www.fiber35diet.com

# References

1. Gill SR, et al., "Metagenomic analysis of the human distal gut microbiome." Science. 2006 Jun 2;312(5778):1355-9.
2. Phillips MR, "Gut reaction; Environmental effects on the human microbiota." Envir Health Perspect. 2009 May;117(5):A198-A205.
3. Penders J, et al., "Factors influencing the composition of the intestinal microbiota in early infancy." Pediatrics. 2006 Aug;118(2):511-21.
4. Mariat D, et al., "The Firmicutes/Bacteriodetes ratio of the human microbiota changes with age." BMC Microbiol. 2009 Jun 9;9:123.
5. Mitsuoka T., "Intestinal flora and human health." Asia Pacific J Clin Nutr. 1996 5(1):2-9.
6. Woodmansey EJ, "Intestinal bacteria and ageing." J Appl Microbiol. 2007 May;102(5):1178-86.
7. Lewis SJ, et al., "The metabolic consequences of slow colonic transit time." Am J Gastroenterol. 1999 Aug;94(8):2010-6.
8. Collins MD and Gibson GR, "Probiotics, prebiotics, and synbiotics: approaches for modulating the microbial ecology of the gut." Am J Clin Nutr. 1999 May;69(5):1052S 1057S.
9. Gorbach SL., "The intestinal microflora and its colon cancer connection." Infection. 1982 Nov-Dec;10(6):379-84.
10. Hawrelak JA and Myers SP, "The causes of intestinal dysbiosis: a review." Alt Med Rev. 2004 9(2):180-96.
11. Cummings JH, et al., "The effect of meat protein and dietary fiber on colonic function and metabolism. Bacterial metabolites in feces and urine." Am J Clin Nutr. 1979 Oct;32(10):2094-101.
12. Macpherson AJ and Uhr T, "Induction of protective IgA by intestinal dendritic cells carrying commensal bacteria." Science. 2004 Mar 12;303(5664):1662-5.
13. Collins SM, "Modulation of intestinal inflammation by stress: basic mechanisms and clinical relevance." Am J Physiol Gastrointest Liver Physiol. 2001 Mar;280(3):G315-8.
14. Nord CE, "The effect of antimicrobial agents on the ecology of the human intestinal microflora." Vet Microbiol. 1993 Jun;35(3-4):193-7.
15. Young VB and Schmidt TM, "Antibiotic-Associated Diarrhea Accompanied by Large Scale Alterations in the Composition of the Fecal Microbiota." J Clin Microbiol. 2004 March; 42(3): 1203–1206.
16. http://www.uptodate.com/contents/patient-information-antibiotic-associated-diarrhea-clostridium-difficile
17. Cremonini F, et al., "Meta-analysis: the effect of probiotic administration on antibiotic-associated diarrhoea." Aliment Pharmacol Ther. 2002; 16:1461–7.
18. Williams NT, "Probiotics." American Journal of Health-System Pharmacy. 2010;67(6):449-458.
19. Amin O, "Seasonal prevalence of intestinal parasites in the United States during 2000." Am J Trop Med Hyg. 2002 Jun;66(6):799-803.
20. http://www.cdc.gov/getsmart/antibiotic-use/anitbiotic-resistance-faqs.html#d
21. Paul IM, et al., "Antibiotic prescribing during pediatric ambulatory care visits for asthma." Pediatrics. 2011 Jun;127(6):1014-21.
22. Compare D, et al., "Effects of long-term PPI treatment on producing bowel symptoms and SIBO." Eur J Clin Invest. 2011 Apr;41(4):380-6.

23. Chey, WD, et al., "Proton pump inhibitors, irritable bowel syndrome, and small intestinal bacterial overgrowth: coincidence or Newton's third law revisited?" Clin Gastroenterol Hepatol. 2010 Jun;8(6):480-2.

24. Dial S, et al., "Proton pump inhibitor use and risk of community-acquired Clostridium difficile-associated disease defined by prescription for oral vancomycin therapy." CMAJ. 2006 Sep 26;175(7):745-8.

25. Martinez AC, et al., " Risk factors for esophageal candidiasis." Eur J Clin Microbiol Infect Dis. 2000 Feb;19(2):96-100.

26. Sarkar, M, et al., "Proton-pump inhibitor use and the risk for community-acquired pneumonia." Ann Intern Med. 2008 Sep 16;149(6):391-8.

27. Tarquonik LE, et al., "Use of proton pump inhibitors and risk of osteoporosis-related fractures." CMAJ. 2008 Aug 12;179(4):319-26.

28. Wright J and Lenard L, *Why Stomach Acid is Good for You.* M Evans and Co, Inc, 2001.

29. http://www.ewg.org/reports/bodyburden2/execsumm.php

30. Fazeli M, et al., "Cadmium chloride exhibits a profound toxic effect on bacterial microflora of the mice gastrointestinal tract." Hum Exp Toxicol. 2011 Feb;30(2):152-9.

31. Bjorkholm B, et al., "Intestinal microbiota regulate xenobiotic metabolism in the liver." PLoS One. 2009 Sep 9;4(9):e6958.

32. http://www.who.int/foodsafety/fs_management/en/probiotic_guidelines.pdf

33. Floch MH and Kim AS, Eds., *Probiotics A Clinical Guide,* SLACK Inc., 2010, p. 141.

34. Borchers A, et al., "Probiotics and immunity." J of Gastroenterol. 2009;44:26-46.

35. Parkes GC, et al., "Treating irritable bowel syndrome with probiotics: the evidence." Proc Nutr Soc. 2010 May;69(2):187-94.

36. Camilleri M, "Probiotics and irritable bowel syndrome: rationale, putative mechanisms, and evidence of clinical efficacy. J Clin Gastroenterol. 2006 Mar;40(3):264-9.

37. Pimentel M, et al., "Eradication of small intestinal bacterial overgrowth reduces symptoms of irritable bowel syndrome." Am J Gastroenterol. 2000 Dec;95(12):3503-6.

38. Williams EA, et al., "Clinical trial: a multistrain probiotic preparation significantly reduces symptoms of irritable bowel syndrome in a double-blind placebo-controlled study." Aliment Pharmacol Ther. 2009 Jan;29(1):97-103.

39. Jarvis WR, et al., "National point prevalence of Clostridium difficile in US health care facility inpatients, 2008." Am J Infect Control. 2009 May;37(4):263-70.

40. McFarland LV, "Meta-analysis of probiotics for the prevention of antibiotic associated diarrhea and the treatment of Clostridium difficile disease." Am J Gastroenterol. 2006 Apr;101(4):812-22.

41. MacFarland LV, "Meta-analysis of probiotics for the prevention of traveler's diarrhea." Travel Med Infect Dis. 2007 Mar;5(2):97-105.

42. Allen SJ, et al., "Probiotics for treating infectious diarrhoea." Cochrane Database Syst Rev. 2004;(2):CD003048.

43. Zoppi G, et al., "The intestinal ecosystem in chronic functional constipation." Acta Paediatr. 1998 Aug;87(8):836-41.

44. Chmielewska A and Szajewska H, "Systematic review of randomised controlled trials: Probiotics for functional constipation." World J Gastroenterol. 2010 January 7; 16(1): 69–75.

45. Salminen S and Salminen E, "Lactulose, lactic acid bacteria, intestinal microecology and mucosal protection." Scand J Gastroenterol Suppl. 1997;222:45-8.

46. Lesbros-Pantoflickova A, et al., "Helicobacter pylori and probiotics." J Nutr. 2007 Mar;137(3 Suppl 2):812S-8S.

47. Isolauri E, et al., "Probiotics: effects on immunity." Am J Clin Nutr. 2001 Feb;73(2 Suppl):444S-450S.
48. Leyer GL, et al., "Probiotic effects on cold and influenza-like symptom incidence and duration in children." Pediatrics. 2009 Aug;124(2):e172-9.
49. Proal AD, et al., "Autoimmune disease in the era of the metagenome." Autoimmun Rev. 2009 Jul;8(8):677-81.
50. Ouwehand AC, "Antiallergic effects of probiotics." J Nutr. 2007 Mar;137 (3 Suppl 2):794S-7S.
51. Weiss ST, "Eat dirt--the hygiene hypothesis and allergic diseases." N Engl J Med. 2002 Sep 19;347(12):930-1.
52. Isolauri E, et al., "Probiotics in the management of atopic eczema." Clin Exp Allergy. 2000 Nov;30(11):1604-10.
53. Kalliomaki M, et al., "Probiotics and prevention of atopic disease: 4-year follow-up of a randomised placebo-controlled trial." Lancet. 2003 May 31;361(9372):1869-71.
54. Reid G, at al., "Oral probiotics can resolve urogenital infections." FEMS Immunol Med Microbiol. 2001 Feb;30(1):49-52.
55. Hilton E, et al., "Ingestion of yogurt containing Lactobacillus acidophilus as prophylaxis for candidal vaginitis." Ann Intern Med. 1992 Mar 1;116(5):353-7.
56. Falagas ME, et al., "Probiotics for prevention of recurrent urinary tract infections in women: a review of the evidence from microbiological and clinical studies." Drugs. 2006;66(9):1253-61.
57. Fendler C, et al., "Frequency of triggering bacteria in patients with reactive arthritis and undifferentiated oligoarthritis and the relative importance of the tests used for diagnosis." Ann Rheum Dis. 2001 Apr;60(4):337-43.
58. Peltonin, et al., "Changes of faecal flora in rheumatoid arthritis during fasting and one-year vegetarian diet." Br J Rheumatol. 1994 Jul;33(7):638-43.
59. Karimi O, et al., "Probiotics (VSL#3) in arthralgia in patients with ulcerative colitis and Crohn's disease: a pilot study." Drugs Today (Barc). 2005 Jul;41(7):453-9.
60. Mandel DR, et al., "Bacillus coagulans: a viable adjunct therapy for relieving symptoms of rheumatoid arthritis according to a randomized, controlled trial." BMC Complement Altern Med. 2010 Jan 12;10:1.
61. Sandek A, et al., "Altered intestinal function in patients with chronic heart failure." J Am Coll Cardiol. 2007 Oct 16;50(16):1561-9.
62. Erridge E, et al., "A high-fat meal induces low-grade endotoxemia: evidence of a novel mechanism of postprandial inflammation." Am J Clin Nutr. 2007 Nov;86(5):1286-92.
63. Cani PD, et al., "Metabolic endotoxemia initiates obesity and insulin resistance." Diabetes. 2007 Jul;56(7):1761-72.
64. Larsen N, et al., "Gut microbiota in human adults with type 2 diabetes differs from non-diabetic adults." PLoS One. 2010 Feb 5;5(2):e9085.
65. Turnbaugh PJ, et al., "An obesity-associated gut microbiome with increased capacity for energy harvest." Nature. 2006 Dec 21;444(7122):1027-31.
66. European Association for the Study of Obesity. "Probiotics May Help Ward Off Obesity, Study In Pregnant Women Suggests." ScienceDaily, 8 May 2009.
67. Maier SF and Watkins LR, "Cytokines for psychologists: implications of bidirectional immune-to-brain communication for understanding behavior, mood, and cognition." Psychol Rev. 1998 Jan;105(1):83-107.
68. Rao AV et al., "Cytokines for psychologists: implications of bidirectional immune-to-brain communication for understanding behavior, mood, and cognition." Gut Pathog. 2009 Mar 19;1(1):6.

# About the Author

**Brenda Watson**, C.N.C., is among the foremost authorities today on natural digestive care and nutrition. A New York Times best-selling author and celebrated PBS mainstay, she began her career in alternative medicine more than a decade ago after her own battle with prolonged illness. Through her clinical work, Brenda discovered the natural remedies that helped her patients improve their health and soon after began formulating her own nutritional digestive blends.

In 1997 Brenda and her husband, Stan Watson, founded Tampa Bay, Florida-based ReNew Life Formulas, Inc. With offices in the U.S. and Canada, the company manufactures and distributes a full line of natural digestive care products and functional foods and reaches more than 3 million people annually through a commitment to retailer and consumer education.

Visit www.brendawatson.com for the latest information on Brenda Watson.